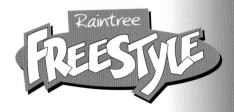

THE ENVIRONMENT CHALLENGE

PROMOTING HEALTH AND PREVENTING DISEASE

Rebecca Vickers

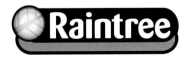

Chicago, Illinois

www.heinemannraintree.com
Visit our website to find out more information about Heinemann-Raintree books.

To order:

☎ Phone 888-454-2279

💻 Visit www.heinemannraintree.com to browse our catalog and order online.

Edited by Andrew Farrow and Adam Miller
Designed by Victoria Allen
Original illustrations © Capstone Global Library Ltd.
Illustrated by Tower Designs UK Limited
Picture research by Mica Brancic
Production by Camilla Cross
Originated by Capstone Global Library Ltd.
Printed and bound in China by South China Printing Company.

15 14 13 12 11
10 9 8 7 6 5 4 3 2 1

Library of Congress Cataloging-in-Publication Data
Vickers, Rebecca.
  Promoting health, preventing disease / Rebecca Vickers.
    p. cm.—(The environment challenge)
  Includes bibliographical references and index.
  ISBN 978-1-4109-4301-9 (hb freestyle)—ISBN 978-1-4109-4308-8 (pb freestyle) 1. Public health—United States. 2. Health promotion—United States. 3. Medicine, Preventive—United States. 4. Self-care, Health—United States. I. Title.
  RA425.V53 2012
  362.1—dc22   2010052726

ISBNs: 978-1-4109-4301-9 (HC); 978-1-4109-4308-8 (PB)

Acknowledgments
The author and publishers are grateful to the following for permission to reproduce copyright material: Alamy p. 23 © Christopher Pillitz; Corbis p. 7 © CARLOS BARRIA/ Reuters, p.15 © Ann Johansson, p. 14 © Ghislain & Marie David de Lossy/cultura, p. 16 © PIYAL ADHIKARY/epa, p. 17 Reuters/© Jonathan Ernst, p. 20 © Ted Horowitz, p. 25 © ANTONY NJUGUNA/Reuters, p. 26 © Michael Ainsworth / Dallas Morning News/, p. 31 Reuters/© Damir Sagolj, p. 32 © Hugh Sitton, p. 34 © Gideon Mendel, p. 35 © Howard Davies, p. 40 © Mika, p. 41 Blend Images/© Dave and Les Jacobs; Getty Images p. 13, p. 4 Iconica/Smith Collection, p. 6 AFP/Jeff Haynes, p. 9 Taxi/Chris Clinton, p. 10 Photodisc/Nick Koudis, p. 11 Photodisc/SMC Images, p. 12 Matt Cardy, p. 19 AFP, p. 21 Justin Sullivan, p. 22 Christopher Pillitz, p. 27 Frank Micelotta, p. 28 AFP/Georges Gobet, p. 29 AFP/Timothy A. Clary, p. 30 AFP/Simon Maina, p. 36 Photodisc/Digital Vision, p. 37 AFP/ Farjana K. Godhuly, p. 38 AFP/Farjana K. Godhuly.

Cover photograph of a Filipino nurse injecting a boy with a measles vaccination in Tondo, Manila, reproduced with permission of Getty Images/AFP photo/Noel Cells.

We would like to thank Michael D. Mastrandrea, Ph.D. for his invaluable help in the preparation of this book.

Every effort has been made to contact copyright holders of any material reproduced in this book. Any omissions will be rectified in subsequent printings if notice is given to the publisher.

Contents

Words appearing in the text in bold, **like this**, are explained in the glossary.

Every Problem Has a Solution

There is a well-known saying that a person can either be a part of the problem or a part of the solution. Of course, everyone would prefer to be part of the solution. But how can that happen? How can you help solve the problems of promoting health and preventing disease throughout the world?

This seems to be a huge, almost overwhelming, challenge. However, like a jigsaw puzzle, lots of the problems in life are best handled by dividing them into smaller, more manageable pieces. It also helps to group related issues together.

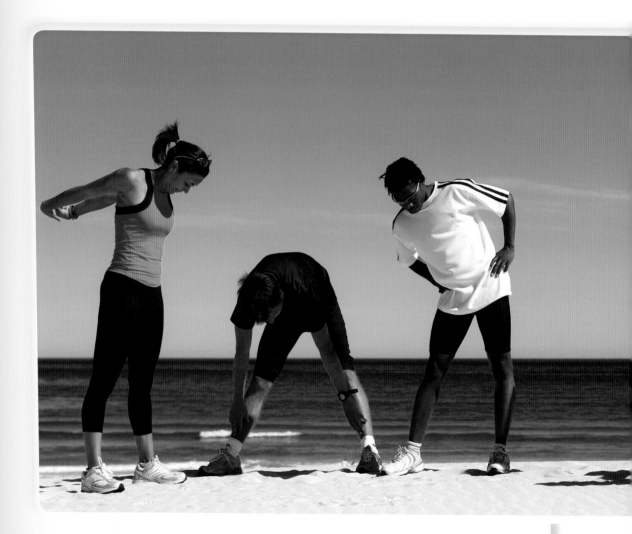

Every person can make a difference to the health of the world by taking responsibility for their own health and physical well-being.

What could be more important than being healthy?

The problems connected to promoting health and preventing disease are among the most important ones facing humankind today. People need to take responsibility for solving these problems in their personal lives, in their neighborhoods and communities, and throughout the wider world. Are you up to the challenge?

"He who has health has hope; and he who has hope has everything."

Arab proverb

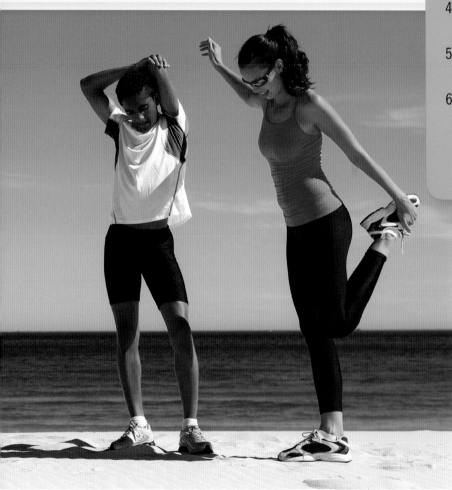

Common steps in problem solving

People have many ideas about the best ways to solve problems, but most agree on the following five key points:

1. Identify the problem.

2. Figure out different ways to solve the problem.

3. Choose the idea that seems to be the best solution.

4. Try to solve the problem using the chosen solution.

5. Evaluate, or judge, the success of your problem solving.

6. Identify unsolved problems, starting the process again.

Bad Habits Equal Bad Health

Medical organizations in many countries around the world are worried about a shocking new fact. At least in **developed countries**, meaning wealthy countries like the United States, it seems likely that the current generation of teenagers will be less healthy than their parents. This will be the first time in recorded history that the health of the new generation is not better than that of the previous generation. How can this have happened? And what can be done about it?

What's the problem?

For young people, there are three main problems causing this health crisis:

- bad eating habits
- the lack of a fitness routine
- bad lifestyle decisions.

But what are the solutions? You need to arm yourself with the knowledge and the determination to tackle these issues in your own life and not be part of the problem!

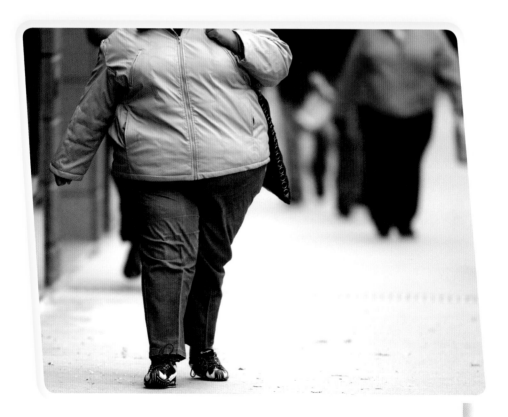

Obesity can cause young people to be tired and breathless.

Food and health

A healthy diet is a good start to a healthy life. To be healthy, eat lots of fruits and vegetables. Also avoid fatty and sugar-loaded foods. Make sure to get enough fiber in your diet. Fiber is a kind of plant material found in grains and in fruits and vegetables.

You've heard all of this before. But why are these things important to maintaining your health?

Making healthy decisions

The human body—especially a young person's body, which is developing into adulthood—needs a variety of vitamins and minerals. Fruits and vegetables are the best sources for many of these essential vitamins and minerals.

Many national governments have lists of what they believe are the minimum daily requirements of vitamins and minerals that the body needs. If you do not get enough of these, your health can suffer. For example, if you do not get enough of the mineral iron, this can lead to anemia. People with anemia do not have enough red blood cells in their bodies, which can make them feel weak and tired. By following recommendations from experts about what to eat, you can meet the challenge to have a healthy body.

In the news

In November 2009, newspapers around the world were full of reports that over one-third of all young people in the United States between the ages of 17 and 24 were not fit enough to serve in the U.S. military. This was usually due to **obesity**, meaning that many kids are very overweight. Curt Gilroy, who works for the U.S. government office in charge of finding new soldiers, said of the problem: "Young people, by and large, can't do push-ups. And they can't do pull-ups. And they can't run."

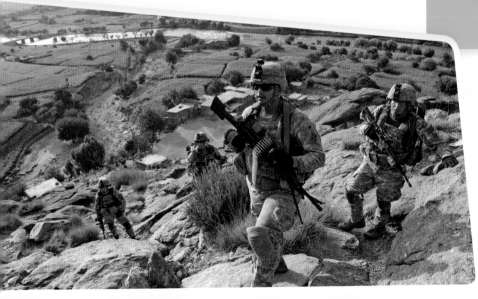

Being a teenage couch potato does not prepare you for life in the military.

How would you choose to get fitter and meet the challenge of promoting your own health and well-being? What if you hate team sports and can't stand running or swimming? Remember that these are not your only choices. Use a Venn diagram like the one shown here to identify the qualities you would like (or would *not* like) to have in an exercise program. See where the overlap occurs, and give some of those forms of exercise a try.

Exercise and fitness

To take control of your own health, it is also important to get regular exercise.

How does exercise keep you healthy?

The human body is made up of body systems that have different functions. Regular exercise can help all the body systems work their best. For example, the cardiovascular system, which involves the heart, the lungs, and the flow of blood around the body, needs the stimulation that regular exercise provides. A well-exercised body is able to carry more oxygen around the body and remove waste from the body.

Endorphins: The feel-good factor

By choosing to exercise, you can maintain and improve the health of your body. But exercise can also make you feel better. This happens in two main ways.

First, regular exercise can give you a feeling of accomplishment. If you exercise by taking part in sports, you can make new friends. Even if you exercise on your own, the improvement in your physical health and appearance can be a real buzz. It can make you feel better about yourself and your life.

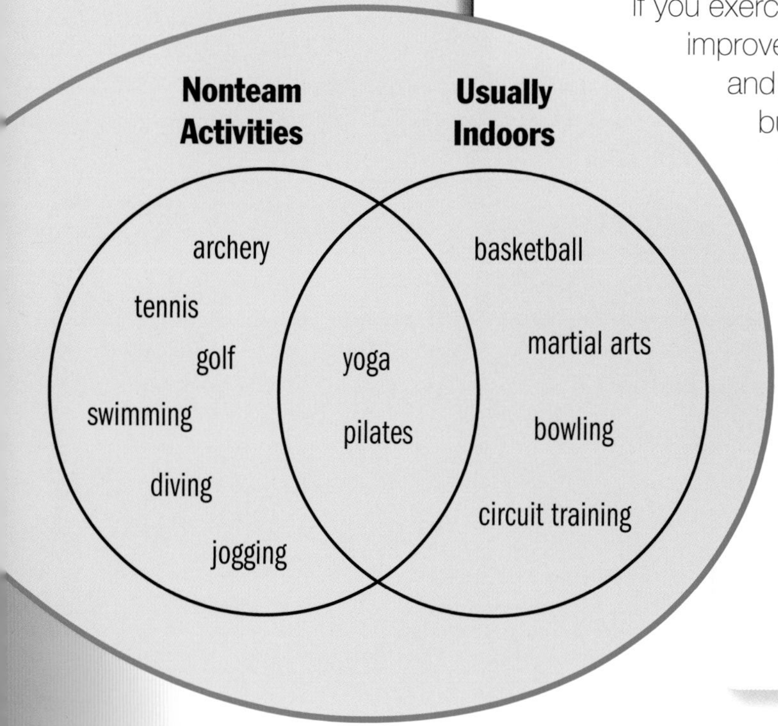

Nonteam Activities / Usually Indoors

archery
tennis
golf
swimming
diving
jogging

yoga
pilates

basketball
martial arts
bowling
circuit training

The activities in the overlap in this Venn diagram are nonteam activities that are usually indoors, yoga and **pilates**.

Second, exercise can make you feel better. This is because physical exercise can stimulate the chemicals in your body. Some of these chemicals, in particular those known as **endorphins**, can make you feel good. The effect of the release of endorphins in the body is sometimes known as the "runner's high." The chemicals adrenaline and dopamine can also be released by the body during exercise and help create a good mood.

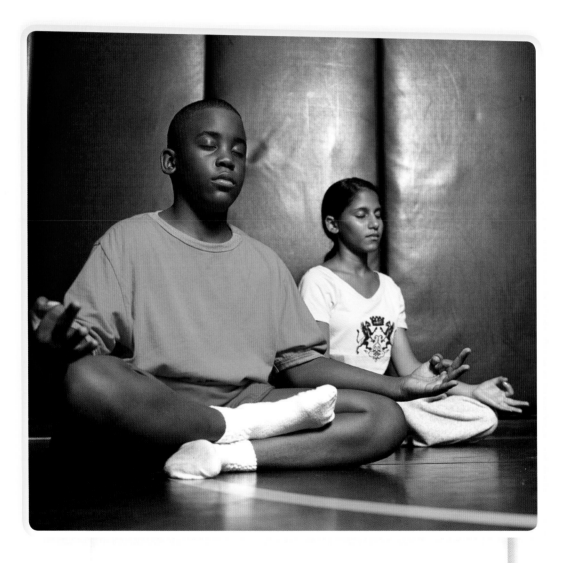

These children are taking part in a school yoga class. There is a form of exercise for everyone. The challenge is finding the one that is best for you.

WORD BANK
endorphins   chemicals in your body that can make you feel good when you exercise
pilates   exercise system that aims to improve strength, flexibility, and posture

Making smart lifestyle decisions

Everything you put in your body has some sort of effect on it. By making wise choices, you can protect and maintain your health. Smoking, using illegal drugs, drinking alcohol, and risky sexual behavior can all damage a person's health.

Smoking is stupid

It has now been over 50 years since the first serious studies linked smoking with diseases and death. So, why does anyone still smoke? Not starting to smoke seems like a no-brainer, but young people still develop this dangerous **addiction**. Almost all new smokers every year are in their mid-teens.

By deciding never to smoke, you will make a huge contribution to your future health. Obviously this will be great for you as an individual. But it is also great for society as a whole. You will never become part of the massive health and financial problems created by the world's one billion smokers.

What would YOU do ?

What can you do to avoid falling into the smoking trap? Think about how you react to the five main ways teens get attracted to this horrible habit:

1. *Experimentation.* The nicotine in tobacco is extremely addictive. What you intend to be an experiment can quickly become a habit that is very hard to break.
2. *Peer pressure.* Remember, if you set your own rules, you don't get swayed by other people's actions.
3. *Rebellion.* Wanting to be cool or rebellious, or to defy adult authority, can be very attractive. But this can backfire. Over two-thirds of the adults who started smoking as teenagers wish they had never started.
4. *Poor self-esteem.* Some young people think that smoking will help them have a better image of themselves, that it will stop them from feeling nervous, or that it might even help them lose weight. None of these things are true. Smoking is known to be bad for the complexion, can make the smoker smell of stale smoke and ash, and has little effect on weight loss.
5. *Home example.* The **statistics** (numbers in studies) say it will be much harder to avoid becoming a smoker if you have close relatives who are already hooked. If one of your parents or an older sibling wants to stop smoking, do everything you can to help them. Get ideas and advice online from www.smokefree.gov.

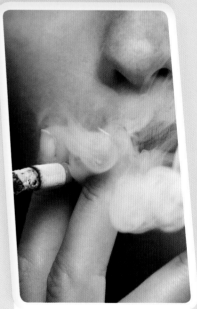

A potentially deadly habit is never cool.

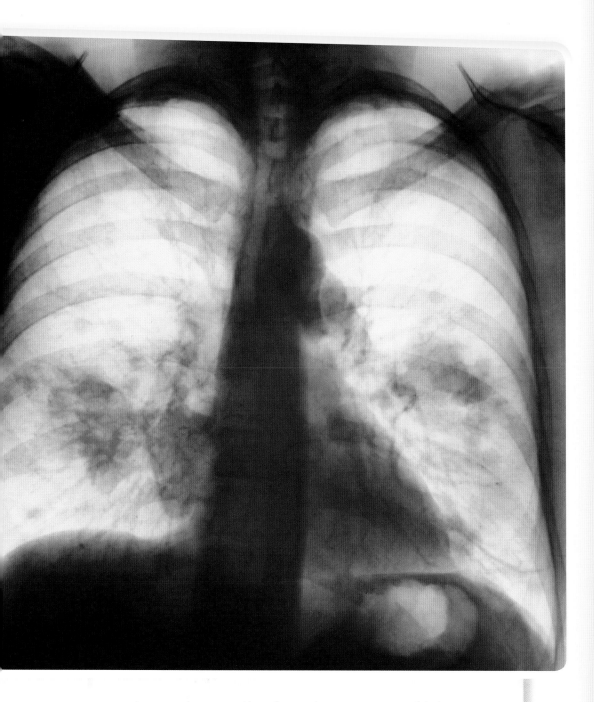

The colored areas on these human lungs are cancer. This is just one of the many health problems caused by smoking.

WORD BANK

addiction   dependence on a habit-causing substance

statistics   collected numbers in studies that can be analyzed to give information about a subject

The long-term social and health problems drug and alcohol abuse cause are huge challenges for individuals and society as a whole. What can you do to help solve these problems? Obviously, deciding not to use illegal drugs or engage in underage drinking is the smart choice. But one of the biggest effects you can have involves alcohol and driving:

- According to the U.S. National Highway Traffic Safety Administration, 26 percent of male drivers between the ages of 15 and 20 who are involved in fatal crashes had been drinking. If you never get in a car with a driver who has been drinking, your risk rate goes down.
- When faced with a potential drunk driver, use peer pressure in a positive way. Let people who have been drinking know how dangerous and stupid you think they are if they try to mix alcohol and driving.

More lifestyle choices to avoid

Smoking isn't the only bad habit that can have a disastrous effect on a person's health. Alcohol abuse, the use of illegal drugs, and the misuse of prescription drugs can also cause severe health damage and even death. Many of the illegal so-called recreational drugs—meaning drugs that people take in social settings, like ecstasy and marijuana—can be highly addictive.

Most alcohol and drug abuse starts in the teenage years. For example, the earlier a person starts drinking alcohol, the more likely he or she is to become a heavy drinker later in life. So, as with smoking, the best health solution is never to let these substances become a problem in the first place.

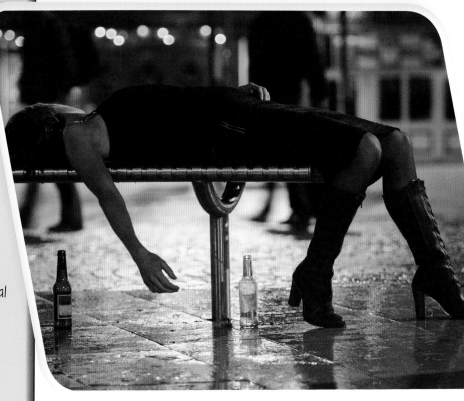

Arm yourself with the facts about underage drinking before making bad choices.

Jamie Oliver's health mission

Sometimes one person with strong views about the solutions to a challenge really can change things. For several years, UK chef Jamie Oliver has been working to educate the public about healthy eating, especially for children. In his 2010 U.S. television series, called *Jamie Oliver's Food Revolution*, Oliver uncovered the poor quality and lack of nutritional value of school meals in the United States. On his show, he tried to show how easy and beneficial it is to cook healthy meals. You can visit Oliver's website to see how he is still working to improve the world's eating habits at www.jamieoliver.com/foundation/.

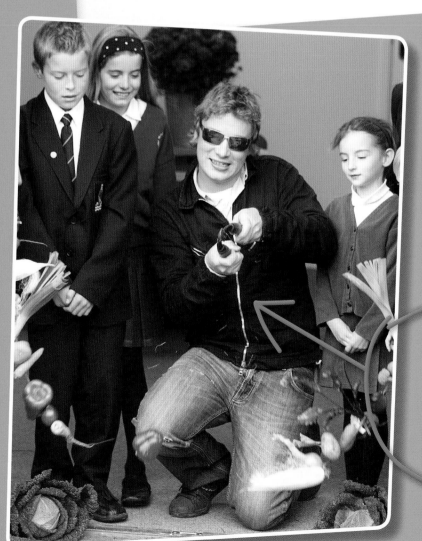

Celebrity chef Jamie Oliver has had to put up with lots of resistance during his international campaign to improve the diets of children.

The Mental Health Challenge

It is easy to recognize physical illnesses in ourselves and our families and friends, but it is harder when the problem relates to mental health. However, particularly in **developed countries**, this is where many major health challenges lie.

Keep your eyes open

Everyone has stresses and strains in their lives. These pressures can be related to schoolwork, bullying, family problems, friendships, or many other things. Eating disorders, self-harming, **depression**, and, in extreme cases, suicide can be the result of pressures that are emotional and **psychological** (relating to the mind).

What would YOU do ?

So, what advice would you give friends or family, or even yourself, if things seem to be getting hard to deal with? Here are a few ideas:

- *Get enough sleep.*
  When you are tired, everything is harder to deal with.
- *Remember to be smart about food and fitness.*
  The same things that keep your body healthy are also good for your mental health.
- *Avoid negative attitudes.*
  A positive outlook can give you hope and confidence.
- *Take time to relax.*
  An overscheduled life can lead to anxiety and no time to think things through.

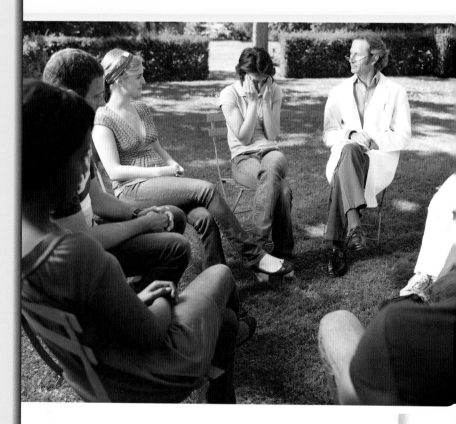

Teenagers are particularly likely to suffer from certain mental health conditions, like depression.

Mental health issues and crime

Recent research shows that large percentages of people in prison, particularly women and young offenders, are suffering from mental disorders. U.S. Department of Justice **statistics** say that more than half of all U.S. prison and jail inmates have mental health problems. So, by paying attention to mental health problems, we could cut the dangers and costs posed to society by crime and the prison system.

A large number of people in prisons and jails have mental health problems. If these disorders were more successfully dealt with, perhaps prison populations wouldn't be so high.

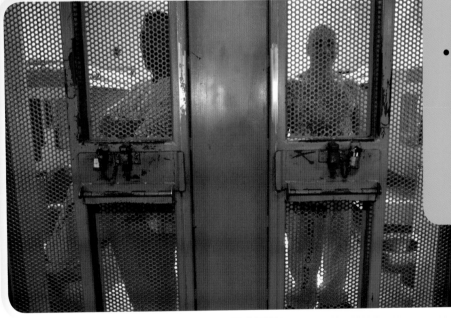

WORD BANK

depression	mental health condition that makes the sufferer feel very sad and hopeless
psychological	related to or affecting the mind
social stigma	something that society sees as a flaw or shortcoming
World Health	United Nations organization that works to solve world health problems

Controlling the Spread of Disease

In many ways, staying healthy and preventing the spread of diseases is easier in the 2000s than ever before. There are more **vaccines** (see box) to help prevent illnesses, more drugs to treat illness, and a better knowledge of **hygiene**, meaning practices that lead to good health. Yet, as people increasingly travel as tourists and move from country to country for work, diseases can spread fast.

What is a vaccine?

A vaccine is a small amount of a disease's infective agent (usually dead or inactive) that is given to a person. This protects the person from catching the disease in the future. The vaccine is usually given as an injection or orally (in the mouth). Some newer vaccines—like a recent one for swine flu—can be inhaled through the nose. (See the vaccine table on page 43.)

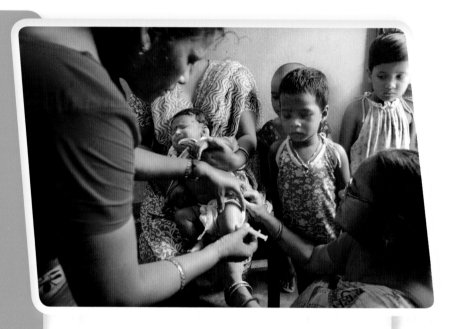

Vaccines are effective at protecting people from some diseases.

Global diseases

Some diseases spread very quickly through groups of people. When this happens in a localized area, it is called an **epidemic**. If it spreads very quickly throughout many countries, it may be declared a **pandemic**.

Pandemics over history include the Black Death in the Middle Ages (the period from roughly the 400s through the 1400s), the Spanish flu just after World War I (1914–18), the sudden spread of **HIV/AIDS** in the 1980s and 1990s (see page 25), and the recent, but less deadly, swine flu pandemic in 2009–2010. Medical experts must rush to develop vaccines and other ways to treat these potentially deadly illnesses.

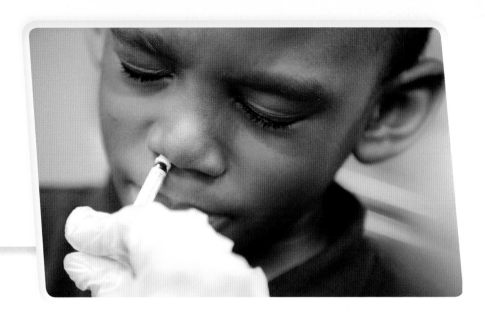

Today, vaccines can be delivered as a nasal spray through the nose. This boy is being given a H1N1 swine flu vaccine.

Smallpox

During the second half of the 1900s, a battle was fought by the **World Health Organization** (**WHO**), medical authorities, and national governments around the world. They wanted to completely end one of the biggest killer diseases of the time: smallpox. This was accomplished by the use of vaccines.

Smallpox had been a major killer for at least 3,000 years. Even though forms of vaccines had been available for over 150 years, the WHO estimated that during the 1900s, three million people annually were still dying from this powerful infection. Something had to be done!

In 1959 the WHO decided to start a major international campaign to rid the world of smallpox through **vaccinations** (giving vaccines). And, only 20 years later, the WHO was able to report that smallpox had been conquered. The last confirmed death was caused by a lab accident in 1978. Read more about this amazing victory at www.who.int/mediacentre/factsheets/smallpox/en/.

The ways diseases spread

Diseases spread in two main ways:

1. *By contagion:* This is the term used to describe the passing of a disease from one person to another. The disease is then referred to as **contagious** or communicable.

2. *Through a recognized disease **vector**:* A vector is the path from one thing to another that a disease agent may follow on its way to infect a human being. For example, the vector for the tropical disease **malaria** is shown below.

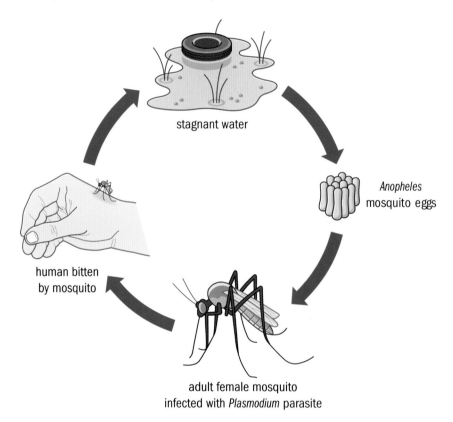

stagnant water

Anopheles mosquito eggs

adult female mosquito infected with *Plasmodium* parasite

human bitten by mosquito

Malaria is not contagious. Everyone who contracts malaria must get a specific parasite that causes the disease from a mosquito bite. Attempts to stop the disease from spreading must be done by breaking or blocking part of the vector.

What is really worrying is the possibility that a **virus** beginning as a vector-spread disease will change, or mutate, into a contagious disease. This happens very rarely, but doctors throughout the world are always on the lookout.

Tracking diseases

Medical scientists called epidemiologists study how diseases are contracted (caught), move, and spread. The **statistics** they collect are used by disease researchers. They can then pinpoint what causes diseases and figure out the best and quickest treatments.

Keeping healthy during Hajj

With people traveling around the world, and with people gathering at huge international events like the Olympic Games and the World Cup, it is easy for disease to spread. So, how do we stop this from happening?

Every year during an annual religious event known as Hajj, over 2.5 million Muslims from more than 70 countries travel at the same time to holy places in Saudi Arabia. Here is some guidance given by medical experts to travelers, to keep them healthy:

- Get a vaccine against meningitis, a sometimes-deadly disease that causes swelling around the brain and spinal cord. The Saudi Ministry of Health requires this.
- Keep clean and be well rested.
- Drink plenty of safe, bottled water, since Saudi Arabia is very hot.
- Take a good first-aid kit and any medications you need to take regularly.
- Eat only fresh, well-cooked food.
- Do not share drinking cups.
- Make sure you have good travel health insurance.

What would YOU do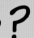

If you were organizing a big event like the Olympic Games, how would you protect the health of those involved? Try using a spider diagram or concept web to brainstorm ideas.

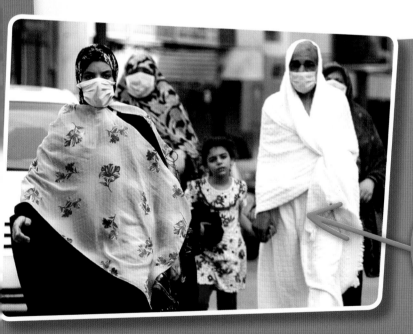

These Muslim Hajj pilgrims are wearing masks to protect them from infection during the 2009 swine flu pandemic.

WORD BANK

contagious capable of being passed from person to person
malaria infectious disease caused by the plasmodium parasite being passed on by a mosquito bite
vector path from one thing to another that a disease agent may follow on its way to infect a human
virus tiny infectious agent that enters living cells, makes copies of itself, and can make a person sick

Bugs without barriers

Infectious diseases (diseases that can spread) do not recognize national boundaries. Neither do the insects and animals that act as vectors for disease. Because of this, the only really effective way to tackle health problems is an international approach. The success of the international campaign against smallpox (see page 17) shows what can be done when people join forces against a disease. But who is leading the fight, and how can you help?

The United Nations' World Health Organization

Since it was founded in 1948, the WHO has worked toward the "attainment by all people of the highest possible level of health." Its recent areas of interest include swine flu, malaria, HIV/AIDS, vaccinations, safe drinking water, healthy eating, and antismoking campaigns. The work of the WHO is paid for by contributions from the United Nations' 193 member countries. You can support the WHO by making sure that others know about the great work it does.

National groups keep countries safe

Most countries have organizations that governments can turn to during an epidemic or pandemic, or during some other public health threat. In the United States, this body is the Centers for Disease Control and Prevention (CDC). The CDC works to prevent and control all infectious diseases. It also provides information and education services relating to public health and workplace health and safety.

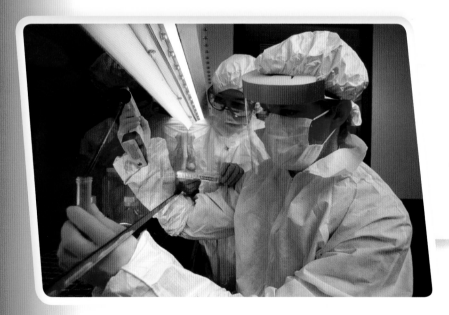

National organizations have to be prepared to contain outbreaks of dangerous diseases.

What would YOU do ?

You may not be able to work on the front lines of disease containment, but everyone can help. A growing problem in our world is the spread of bedbugs. These tiny bugs can make a home in places like beds, and their bites can be very itchy. So, how do you make sure that you sleep tight and don't let the bedbugs bite?:

- In a hotel, don't put your suitcase on the bed or floor.
- Check the bed for bedbug signs. These can be tiny brown marks or blood smears, or even small brownish-orange bugs.
- Hang up clothes rather than using drawers that might have bedbugs.
- When you come home from a trip, wash and dry your clothes at hot temperatures. This will kill most bedbugs and their eggs.
- Don't unpack on the bed or bedroom floor.
- Finally, vacuum out your suitcases and store them away from bedrooms and living areas—never under the bed!

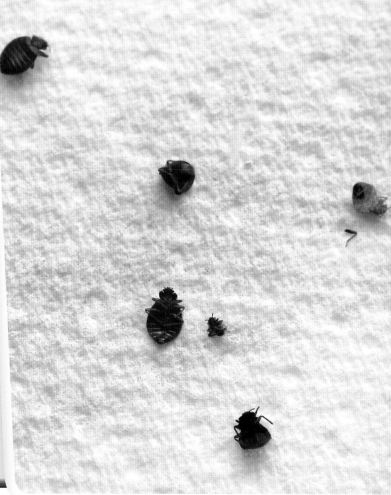

Bedbugs are very hard to get rid of!

ANK
s   capab

Poverty and Health

Wherever there is poverty, there is also an increase in health problems and disease. There is also lower **life expectancy**, meaning the numbers of years a person is expected to live (see the table on page 43). So, figuring out how to deal with poverty and its causes is a step toward making the world a healthier place.

Basic human needs

People living in poverty often lack basic human needs. Here are some of the things identified as being necessary for a healthy physical and mental life:

- adequate housing

- enough food and clean water

- **sanitation** (procedures, such as removing garbage, that lead to good health)

- safety.

Solving the cycle of poverty and its accompanying health problems begins with making sure people have these basic human needs.

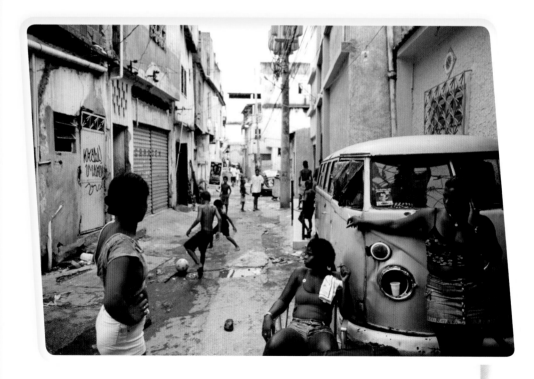

No matter how hard the residents of this slum in Brazil try, bad housing conditions and poor sanitation mean that staying healthy is almost impossible.

Kids suffer the most

When it comes to the effects of poverty, kids are usually hit the hardest. Bad housing conditions, inadequate food, and poor **hygiene** can lower the body's ability to fight illnesses. A poor diet and poor sleeping conditions can also affect a child's education, leading to tiredness and time off school because of illness. **Statistics** from researchers point to a strong link between poverty and poor academic progress.

Levels of child poverty are falling in some **developed countries**. Surprisingly, however, they are rising in other developed countries, and stubbornly staying the same in others.

In the news

In June 2010, *USA Today* reported statistics showing that child poverty in the United States had risen to 22 percent (around 20 million children). This is the highest level in 20 years. Figures also indicate that over 7 million U.S. kids live in extreme poverty, with as many as 8 million children living in homes with no stable source of food. And this poverty is in a country that is more economically developed than almost all others in the world.

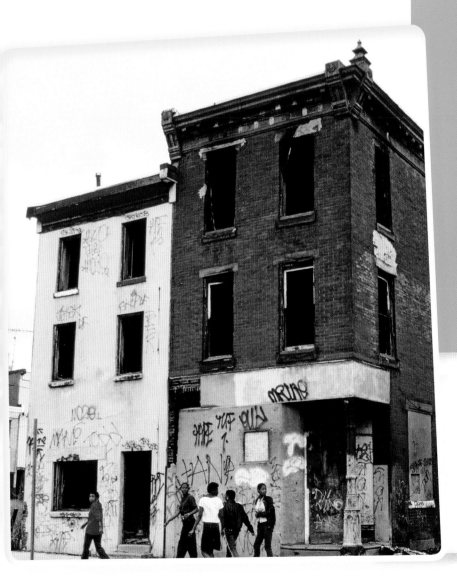

Many developed countries have surprisingly high levels of child poverty. This run-down urban area is in west North Philadelphia.

WORD BANK
life expectancy   number of years a person is expected to live
sanitation   procedures, such as removing sewage and other waste, to protect health

23

Getting help to where it's needed

People living in poverty in **developing countries** (poorer countries) often live in alarming conditions. However, great steps are being made by national governments, with the support of charities and aid agencies.

The United Nations' International Children's Fund (UNICEF), the **WHO**, Oxfam, the Save the Children Fund, and other international charities all support health programs in developing countries. They provide basic health care, clean water, **vaccinations**, and medical supplies. The most successful programs work closely with local people. By training those in the community, charities and aid agencies **empower** local people to improve their own health.

The HIV/AIDS pandemic

During the last 20 years, the spread of the **HIV/AIDS pandemic** has raised health challenges throughout the world. The Human Immunodeficiency **Virus** (HIV) has no known cure, and it leads to a group of deadly diseases. From the time it was first recognized in the early 1980s, it has killed over 25 million people worldwide. Today, more than 33 million people around the globe are infected.

In richer countries, the drugs that help slow down the disease are expensive, but widely available. In poorer countries, this is not the case—but it is improving. With over two million people a year dying of this incurable disease, preventing more infection seems the best solution.

What would YOU do?

Think about the best ways to solve the HIV/AIDS pandemic. Make a table with two columns, labeled "Transmission" and "Prevention," and research the best ways to stop more people from becoming infected. Check out ideas at www.avert.org/prevent-hiv.htm and http://kidshealth.org/kid/health_problems/infection/hiv.html.

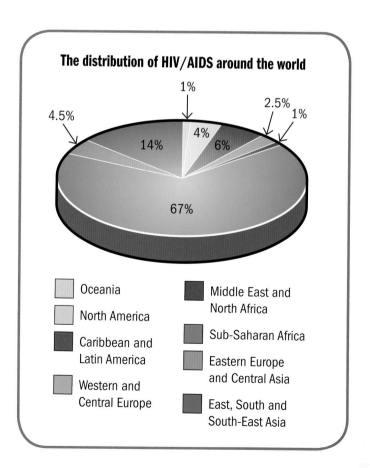

The distribution of HIV/AIDS around the world

1%
2.5%
1%
4.5%
4%
14%
6%
67%

Oceania

North America

Caribbean and Latin America

Western and Central Europe

Middle East and North Africa

Sub-Saharan Africa

Eastern Europe and Central Asia

East, South and South-East Asia

The AMREF method

The African Medical Research Foundation (AMREF) is involved in many projects in the most poverty-stricken parts of Africa. But its workers do not just appear, perform operations and provide vaccinations, and then leave. Rather, many of its projects focus on using the best resource there is in a local community—the people themselves.

By doing this, they create a health care **infrastructure**, or organizational framework. When AMREF forms a health care system at a local level, this local system helps deal with the community's health needs over time. The focus on training local people also means that the traditional medical helpers in a local area, such as the healers and midwives, are part of the system.

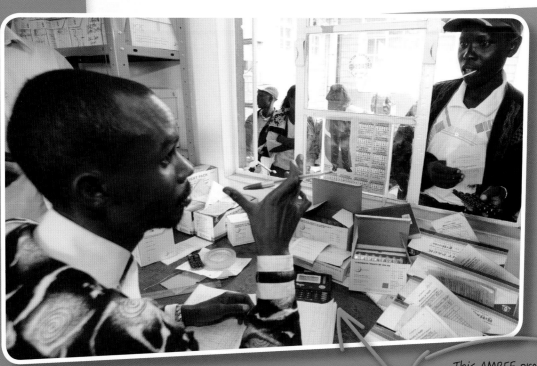

This AMREF project trains local community members to be part of a health care program.

Natural disasters and health

In many ways, the Earth we live on is an unstable and dangerous home. Bad weather, floods, volcanoes, and earthquakes are all able to cause death, destruction, and homelessness. They can also cause the conditions that lead to major health crises. But what if a country hit by a natural disaster is poor and has a weak infrastructure? Then things can get very bad very quickly.

Many developing countries find it difficult to pay for the kind of things that people in developed countries take for granted. This can lead to poor-quality roads, hospitals, power supplies, emergency services, public sanitation, and safe water supplies. A lack of any of these can be annoying and inconvenient when there are no other problems. But, if disaster strikes, these failings quickly lead to health emergencies.

When Hurricane Katrina hit New Orleans in 2005, it was clear that the city was not prepared to take care of those left without shelter, food, and water. These people are waiting in line for a bus to take them from the filthy conditions of the New Orleans Superdome to the better-equipped Astrodome in Houston, Texas.

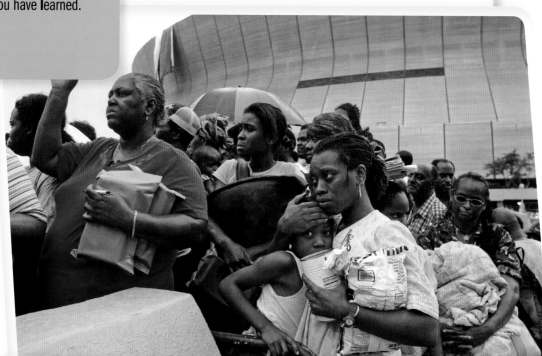

The January 2010 Haiti earthquake

The Caribbean country of Haiti is one of the poorest nations on Earth. Life expectancy is only 61 years. Eighty percent of the population lives in poverty. It has a high rate of **infant mortality** (death of babies under one year old), a high number of AIDS deaths, and lots of problems with violence. Government infrastructure is not very developed, and there is not much financial support for education. It is just the kind of place to find recovery from a natural disaster difficult.

In January 2010, a massive earthquake struck Haiti. After the earthquake hit, international bodies, aid agencies, and national governments all came to Haiti's assistance. The death toll from the earthquake is believed to be around 230,000, but the risk of major disease outbreaks was avoided. However, there were outbreaks of cholera later in the year, after heavy rain during Hurricane Thomas created ideal conditions for the disease.

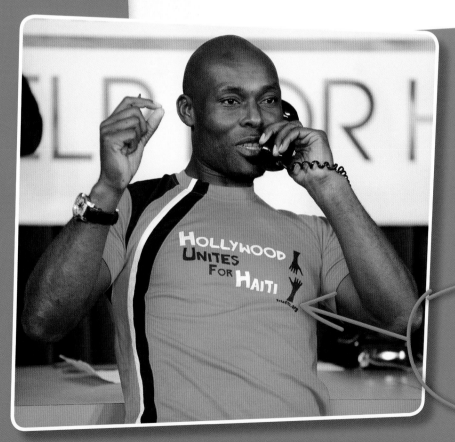

Events like this telethon for the victims of the 2010 Haiti earthquake raise money to help the people hit by natural disasters.

War and Conflict

Poverty and natural disasters are not the only health challenges the world has to face. War and political conflict also put health at risk. For those who fight, war can cause death, injuries, and permanent disabilities.

CASE STUDY

Damaged young warriors

It has been recognized since World War I that soldiers often become **psychologically** damaged because of the horrors they see during war. The condition then known as shell shock is now called post-traumatic stress disorder. The condition can lead to problems with relationships, **depression**, sleep, and anger.

For many years during civil war in Uganda, in Africa, children were kidnapped and forced to fight. These children were treated brutally and expected to treat others brutally. In some cases, they were forced to become addicted to drugs. Now many programs are helping them overcome the horrors they experienced. Find out more about what is being done to help child soldiers at www.child-soldier.org.

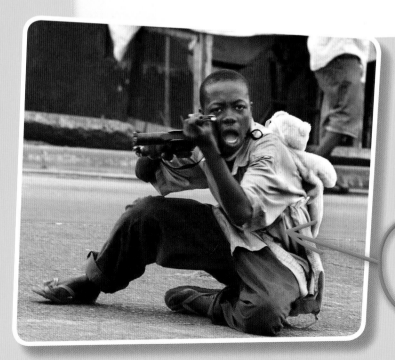

Special camps have now been set up to help and "deprogram" child soldiers like this one.

Victims of war

During wars and conflicts, local people are also affected. They can be caught in the crossfire. And sometimes they are forced from their homes. These victims of war usually find themselves living in overcrowded places with poor or nonexistent clean water and **sanitation**. They may have little or no shelter. In addition to dealing with emotional stress, they are exposed to the spread of disease. **Malnutrition**, a condition caused by a lack of healthy food, is also common.

Helping refugees and displaced persons

But there are people trying to help victims of war. The United Nations' High Commission for **Refugees** (UNHCR) is currently helping over 34 million refugees (people fleeing their homes) and displaced persons around the world. With the money it receives from United Nations member countries, it sets up camps and tries to help refugees return home. Charities like the International Committee of the Red Cross and Doctors Without Borders also supply health professionals to work in refugee camps.

What would YOU do ?

Getting people to talk and to make compromises is easier to say than to do. International organizations and **diplomats** (government representatives) try to maintain good relationships. Are they trying hard enough? What else do you think they could do?

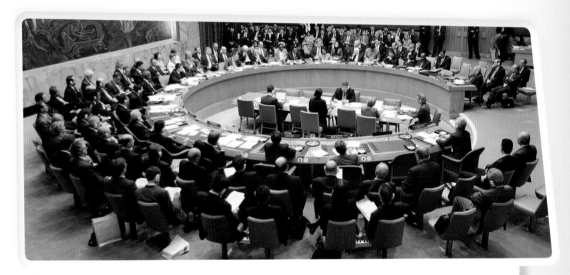

These country representatives at the United Nations are trying to prevent war and conflict. Their success can protect the health and safety of many people.

Health and Our Changing Environment

When we consider our health and the environment, we think about things like the risk of skin cancer from too much exposure to the Sun. But will **climate change** cause more health challenges?

More heat, more water

Statistics show that Earth is getting warmer. This has many consequences. Weather conditions can become more extreme. Warming can lead to icecaps melting, causing sea levels to rise. Flooding, stronger and longer hurricane seasons, and dangerously high temperatures are predicted to become more common over time.

There could be many health effects from these changes. More weather disasters could cause deaths and destroy homes and livelihoods. In some countries, food and clean water supplies could be ruined or difficult to reach.

Governments and international organizations are already making plans. The charity WaterAid has been at the forefront of efforts to protect safe water and improve **sanitation** in countries most at risk. Learn more about its work at www.wateraidamerica.org.

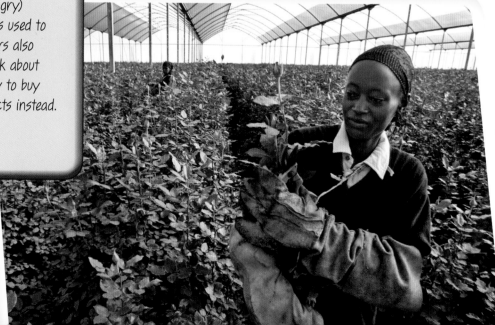

Will malaria spread?

Malaria (see page 18) occurs regularly in tropical and subtropical areas of the world, where 50 percent of Earth's people live. All of them are at risk of this mosquito-borne disease. Some experts think that as the world warms, the type of mosquito that hosts the malaria parasite will move into new areas. Southern Europe, parts of North America, and Australia are all at risk.

Medical researchers are already spending lots of time and money on finding a **vaccine** or better treatments for malaria. So far they have been unsuccessful. With over 350 million people a year getting malaria and nearly 3 million dying, malaria is the world's biggest killer disease. Are we doing enough to stop it?

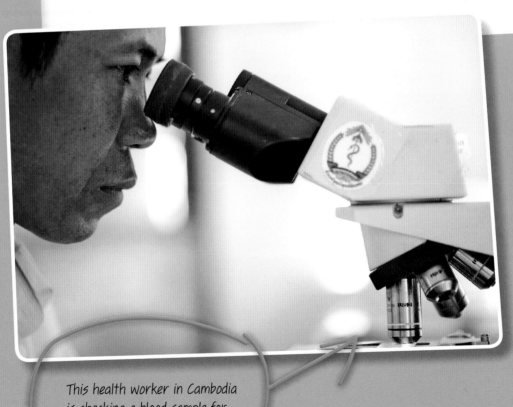

This health worker in Cambodia is checking a blood sample for signs of malaria.

Women Are the Key

All of the people involved in promoting world health agree that women play a very important role in improving the situation. This is true in every part of the world.

Why are women so important?

It is not hard to understand why women are so important for everyone's health. There are physical, traditional, and continuing cultural reasons why this is the case.

Women carry and give birth to the next generation

As the person who carries a child and then gives birth, a woman's knowledge of good health practices is very important. This is true both for her own health as well as for that of her child. In fact, the health of a child starts even before a woman becomes pregnant. If a woman does not have proper nutrition, she might even find it hard to become pregnant in the first place. It becomes even more essential once a woman is carrying a child. Look at some of the fact and figures at www.everymothercounts.org.

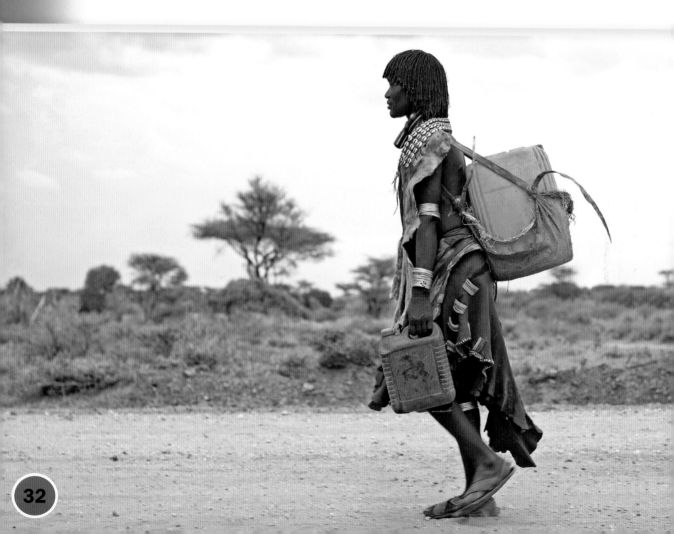

Women are the first educators

As the first educator of a young child, what the mother says, or how she does things herself, is essential to the health and survival of her children. The health knowledge of the mother is passed on to her children in the things she teaches, such as the need for the child to wash his or her hands after using the toilet. Children follow their mothers' examples. These could be positive things like eating healthily, or negative things like smoking.

Women take the lead in nutrition and hygiene

Even in cultures where women have no power, the important aspects of life that relate to food, nutrition, and family **hygiene** almost always fall to the women. In some countries, this extends to growing, harvesting, and storing the food. In fact, throughout the world, between 60 and 80 percent of the farmers are women.

In terms of hygiene, outside of **developed countries**, **rural** women (women who live in the countryside) on average walk 8 kilometers (5 miles) a day, collecting water for household and farming purposes. In parts of rural Africa, it is more like 16 kilometers (10 miles). Clean water is essential to a family's health.

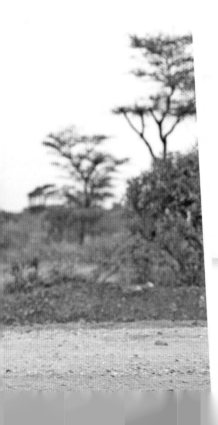

This woman in Ethiopia is walking from her nearest water supply. Many countries do not have piped or even well water in their rural areas.

Making it better and easier

By helping women learn about the best ways to keep themselves and their families healthy, lives will be saved, and people's quality of life will improve.

For example, charity and aid groups often dig wells in impoverished areas. These provide clean water near where people live and grow crops. This gives women much more time to work on their farms and teach their children.

Reproductive choice works

Many women around the world do not have access to good health care during pregnancy and childbirth. These women also do not have birth control supplies or information easily available. These options would allow them to limit the size of their families, or to space out the children they do have. This means they would have more time and money for each child, improving his or her quality of life.

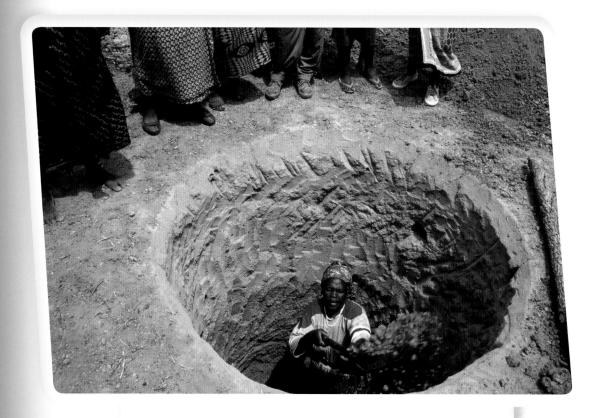

Having a safe, local water supply, like this new well in Zambia, Africa, improves the health and quality of life of the people who live nearby.

Focusing on educating girls

Currently, of the 110 million children around the world who do not receive any education, two-thirds are girls. So, if women are the key to improving and protecting the health of the world, then changing this situation is essential. In many **developing countries**, particularly in rural areas, cultural attitudes toward educating girls need to change. If people are allowed a good education as children, then the possibilities for improving their lives and their families' lives are limitless.

CASE STUDY

Kerala, India

For 50 years, the state of Kerala, in India, has championed the education of girls. In India as a whole, only half of women are able to read and write. In Kerala, 90 percent of women can read, and all girls under 14 are required to go to school. So, has this improved health? Yes!

Kerala is not a wealthy state, but it has the best **statistics** in India for maternal (mother) and child health. And, Kerala has an **infant mortality** rate that is less than one-quarter of the average for India. A United Nations Food and Agriculture Organization report states that the "Kerala example" of educating girls has done more to fight hunger and **malnutrition** than any other efforts.

> "Investing in girls is the right thing to do. It is also the smart thing to do."
>
> Ngozi Okonjo-Iweala, managing director, the World Bank, 2009

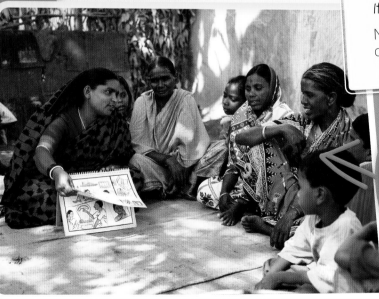

This health instructor in rural India is using an illustrated visual aid to help a group of women and children understand what they can do to keep from getting **malaria**.

Mothers' money and health

Throughout the developing countries of the world, it has been shown that 90 percent of the money that a mother makes is spent on her family. But only about 25 to 30 percent of the money earned by a father comes back to the family. Other statistics show that a woman who earns and has control over her own money will be healthier herself and have healthier children.

Microfinancing and health

In most of the poorer parts of the world, women cannot get loans to set up businesses or improve their farms. This is because they do not own anything that they can use as collateral, meaning something of value that secures the loan.

For the last 30 years, various programs have given loans to women who otherwise would not have been able to secure them. These programs are known as **microfinance** or microcredit. Places with well-developed programs like this have given many women the chance to take control of their lives and improve the health of their families.

Throughout the world, women can make a huge difference to the lives of their children.

Bangladesh's Grameen Bank

For over 30 years, the Grameen Bank, a microfinancing business, has given small loans to poor women in the South Asian country of Bangladesh. Since it started in the mid-1970s, it has loaned out over $6.5 billion. In 2006 the bank and its founder, Muhammad Yunus, were awarded the Nobel Peace Prize. It is the only business to ever receive this important international award. One of the unique things about the Grameen Bank is that all of the women it lends to are required to sign the bank's mission statement, known as the "16 Decisions." Many of these "16 Decisions" relate to the need to protect and promote health. Here are a few:

- Live in well-repaired and maintained houses.

- Grow and eat plenty of vegetables.

- Keep your family small.

- Educate your children.

- Keep your children and their environment clean.

- Look after your health.

- Build and use proper **sanitation**.

- Use only clean water.

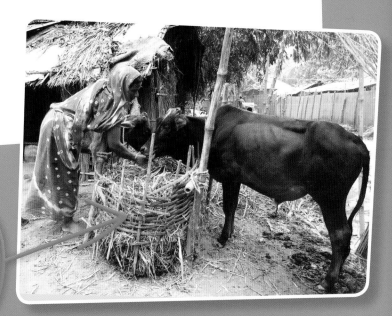

This woman in Bangladesh is feeding the cattle she bought with a loan from the Grameen Bank. When women earn and control their own money, both they and their children are healthier.

Looking to the Future

The issue of promoting health and preventing disease can be approached in many ways. It can be as simple as deciding to eat your fruits and vegetables every day, or as difficult as solving **climate change** or the effects of poverty! There is not just one problem that needs solving, but rather thousands of different ones that all need special attention.

Actions have consequences

Many of the actions we take in our lives can have effects on health. For example, we all know that alcohol abuse can have terrible effects on individuals and on their families. But it can also have a much bigger impact on the society we live in. The most recent figures from the National Institute on Drug Abuse show the cost of alcohol abuse to U.S. society is $185 billion a year in medical bills, crime, and loss of work.

There are other ways in which our actions can have unimagined consequences. For example, a lot of research time and money has been spent developing and promoting the use of ethanol. This is a plant-based vehicle fuel that is renewable. This means it is capable of being reused— unlike gasoline, which cannot be reused. Sounds like a great idea, doesn't it?

However, it gets complicated. To make money, some farmers in South America are now growing crops of soybeans, which can be used to make ethanol. This means they do not grow food crops for local people, since this earns less. Rain forest areas have also been cleared for ethanol crops. This is a problem, as rain forests help keep the world's climate stable. Ideas like these seem straightforward, but the realities are never that simple.

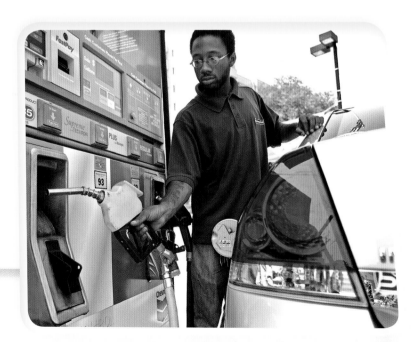

Various laws in the United States encourage the production and use of ethanol because it is a cheaper, green fuel.

Cocaine consequences

People from wealthier parts of the world who use drugs like heroin and cocaine think they are only having an effect on their own health. They are wrong. For example, in cocaine-supplying countries—like Colombia in South America, shown here—there are many negative side effects of the drug trade.

Workers spend their time growing, harvesting, and processing the illegal drugs. Food crops take second place because they are not worth as much. As a result, local people may go hungry. Many of those involved in the drug trade get addicted to the drug crops with which they work. Violent criminal gangs become as powerful as governments, but usually make no financial contribution to the **infrastructure** of the country.

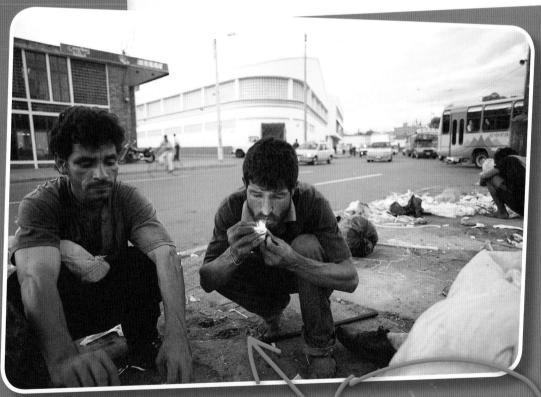

In Bogota, Columbia, thousands of drug addicts live on the streets in harsh conditions.

Working for change

If you want to really get involved and help meet the health challenges of the future, you can think now about different careers you could consider. Here are some ideas:

- *Pursue medical and health-related careers.*
  From being a doctor, to a dentist, to a midwife, there are medical careers at all levels that you can train for. Once you are qualified, you can work in your own community or help with the promotion of health and disease prevention around the world.

- *Research your way to answers.*
  Many of the health problems in the world need specific answers. Doing scientific and **statistical** research can be the path to finding new approaches, cures, and treatments.

- *Keep the problems from starting.*
  You could work in local, national, and international government organizations, or be a **diplomat**. That way you could be part of the "talking shops" that help prevent health problems from happening in the first place. Supporting the infrastructure of society can also provide help when natural or human-created disasters occur.

Apart from jobs, everyone can support the challenge of promoting health and preventing disease by volunteering or giving money to international organizations and aid agencies around the world. We can all make a difference!

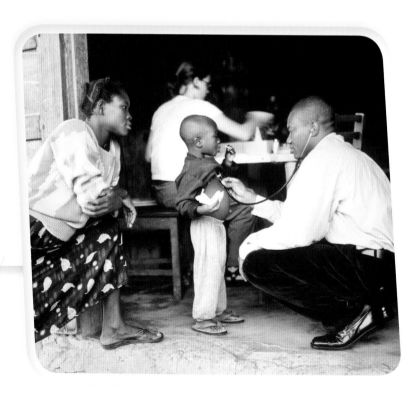

This doctor is treating a child in Ghana. Many doctors and medical students volunteer their vacation time to help poor people in **rural** areas of Africa.

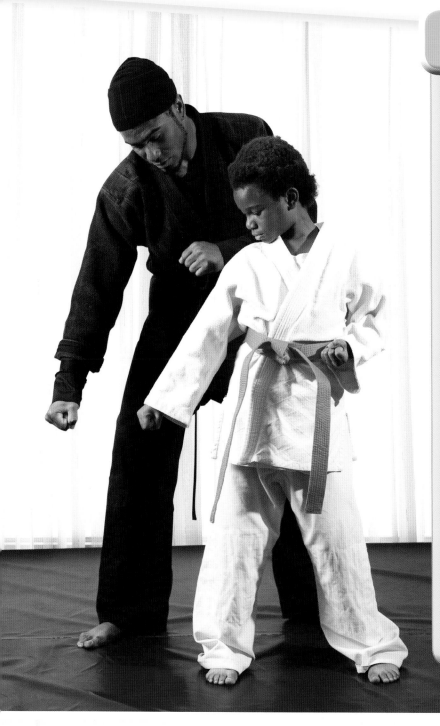

 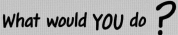
Here is a suggested "top five" list of things that can be done to meet the challenge of promoting health and preventing disease:

1. Educate and **empower** women.
2. Take responsibility for your own physical and mental health.
3. Help friends and relatives to make good choices about their health and well-being.
4. Support your local community, and society more generally, in attempts to prevent the spread of diseases and bad lifestyle choices.
5. Use your time to get involved as a volunteer in activities that promote health.

Do you agree that these are the top five? What other things do you think could be solutions to the health challenge? Brainstorm your ideas on a concept web, or make this top five into a "top 10" list.

By doing simple things, like helping others to get fit, you can play your part in making the world a healthier place.

Fact File

Keeping babies alive

This list shows **infant mortality** for a selection of countries. Infant mortality is the proportion of babies born who die before they reach one year old.

Rank	Country	Deaths per 1000 births
1	Angola	180.21
6	Somalia	109.19
11	Nigeria	94.35
21	Laos	77.76
28	Pakistan	67.36
37	Haiti	59.69
51	India	50.78
61	South Africa	44.42
78	Peru	28.62
110	Mexico	18.42
113	China	20.25
152	Russia	10.56
180	United States	6.22
190	Canada	5.04
194	United Kingdom	4.85
195	Australia	4.67
217	France	3.33
221	Japan	2.79
222	Sweden	2.75
224	Singapore	2.31

source: estimated 2010 figures from the CIA World Factbook

Diseases protected against by vaccines:

The following list shows some of the most widespread major diseases for which there are **vaccines**. Vaccines can protect against diseases caused by both viruses and bacteria.

Viral infections:	Bacterial infections:
Hepatitis A	Anthrax
Hepatitis B	Diphtheria
Influenza	Haemophilus Influenzae b (Hib)
Japanese B encephalitis	Meningococcal meningitis
Measles	Pertussis (whooping cough)
Mumps	Pneumococcal pneumonia
Polio	Tetanus
Rabies	Tuberculosis (BCG)
Rubella	Typhoid
Tick-borne encephalitis	
Yellow fever	

The national life lottery

This list shows **life expectancy** at birth for a selection of countries.

Rank	Country	Years
1	Macau	84.36
3	Japan	82.12
6	Australia	81.63
17	New Zealand	80.36
30	Netherlands	79.40
32	Germany	79.26
36	United Kingdom	79.01
46	Ireland	78.24
49	United States	78.11
66	Argentina	76.56
71	Mexico	76.06
107	Jamaica	73.53
108	China	73.47
137	Indonesia	70.76
161	India	66.09
170	North Korea	63.81
208	Sudan	51.42

source: estimated 2010 figures from the CIA World Factbook

Glossary

addiction dependence on a habit-forming substance

climate change changes to nature's weather patterns over time, possibly because of human actions

contagious capable of being passed from person to person

depression mental health condition that makes the sufferer feel very sad and hopeless

developed country wealthy country where people have a high standard of living

developing country poor country where people do not have a high standard of living

diplomat representative of a national government who helps maintain good relationships with other countries

empower enable or give the ability to do something

endorphins chemicals in your body that can make you feel good after exercise

epidemic spread of a disease in a localized area

HIV/AIDS incurable virus and the group of diseases it causes. "HIV" stands for "Human Immunodeficiency Virus." "AIDS" stands for "Acquired Immune Deficiency Syndrome."

hygiene cleanliness practices that lead to good health

infant mortality death of babies under the age of one year

infectious capable of spreading and being caught by others

infrastructure basic organizational framework of a system

life expectancy number of years a person is expected to live

malaria infectious disease caused by the plasmodium parasite being passed on by a mosquito bite. Symptoms include fever and chills.

malnutrition condition caused by a lack of correct amounts of healthy food

microfinance supply of small loans to people who could otherwise not borrow money

obesity being very overweight

pandemic spread of a disease throughout many countries

pilates exercise system that aims to improve strength, flexibility, and posture

psychological related to or affecting the mind

refugee person who flees his or her home because of something like a disaster or war

rural from the countryside

sanitation procedures, such as removing sewage and other waste, to protect health

social stigma something that society sees as a flaw or shortcoming

statistics collected numbers in studies that can be analyzed to give information about a subject

vaccination introduction into the body of inactive disease material, which makes the body produce antibodies to protect itself against getting the disease

vaccine inactive disease material given to a person to make the body produce antibodies, which protect the body from getting the disease

vector path from one thing to another that a disease agent may follow on its way to infect a human being

virus tiny infectious agent that enters living cells, makes copies of itself, and can make a person sick

World Health Organization (WHO) United Nations organization that works to solve world health problems

Find Out More

Books

Bingham, Jane. *Smoking (What's the Deal?)*. Chicago: Heinemann Library, 2006.

Lewis, Barbara A. *The Teen Guide to Global Action*. Minneapolis: Free Spirit, 2008.

Parker, Steve. *Feel Good, Look Great (Life Skills)*. Chicago: Heinemann Library, 2009.

Savage, Lorraine. *Mental Illness (Issues That Concern You)*. Detroit: Greenhaven, 2009.

Sheen, Barbara. *Girls' Guide to Feeling Fabulous (Life Skills)*. Chicago: Heinemann Library, 2009.

Shuster, Kate. *Can Earth Support Our Growing Population? (What Do You Think?)*. Chicago: Heinemann Library, 2009.

Snedden, Robert. *Fighting Infectious Diseases (Microlife)*. Chicago: Heinemann Library, 2007.

Vickers, Rebecca. *Medicine (From Fail to Win!)*. Chicago: Raintree, 2011.

Websites

www.fda.gov
This is the website of the U.S. Food and Drug Administration. Check out this site for information on good food choices and dietary requirements.

www.oxfamamerica.org
This website of the aid agency Oxfam will give you information on its projects worldwide, including up-to-date information on progress in Haiti.

www.un.org/en/
This United Nations website can give you access to information on many global health issues.

Movies

Andromeda Strain (1971).
This thriller is about scientists working against the clock to stop the spread of a deadly infection.

Life, Above All (2010).
This tells the story of a mother and daughter in an HIV/AIDS-stricken community in South Africa.

Documentary films

An Inconvenient Truth (2006).
This film follows former U.S. Vice-President Al Gore's attempts to educate people about global warming.

Malaria, the Serial Killer (2008).
This 52-minute documentary explores the deadly disease malaria.

No Woman, No Cry (2010).
This movie documents the many unnecessary maternal deaths that occur worldwide during childbirth.

Further research

You can do further research on many topics related to the promotion of health and the prevention of disease worldwide. Here are a few ideas:

- asthma
- swine flu
- "superfoods"
- nut allergies
- gene patents
- psychological effects of war
- gender equality
- cash crops
- maternal health.

Index